Baking Soda Power!
Frugal and Natural: Health, Cleaning, and Hygiene Secrets of Baking Soda
2ND EDITION!

By Patty Korman

Table of Contents

Baking Soda Power! Frugal and Natural: Health, Cleaning, and Hygiene Secrets of Baking Soda
Table of Contents
Introduction.
1. Baking soda basics.

    Origins
    Just how does baking soda work?

2. Kitchen cleaning with baking soda.

    Bug repellent
    Odor-killer
    Fridge freshener
    Shiny surfaces
    De-odorizing bottles and flasks
    De-odorizing hands
    Dish soap
    De-odorizing sponges
    Cleaning the microwave and oven
    Mop cleaner
    Better dish soap

3. Cooking with baking soda.

    Reduce acidity in food.
    De-odorizing meat
    Fluffy omelets
    Easier hardboiled eggs
    De-feathering game
    Homemade Gatorade

Substitute for baking powder
  Tenderize meat
  Clean burned pans

4. Bathroom upkeep with baking soda.

    Shower curtains
    Unclogging drains
    Stained toilet
    Glass cleaner
    Bathroom de-odorizing
    Floor, bathtub cleaner
    Toothbrush and comb freshener
    Unclog showerhead
    Natural grout cleaner

5. Laundry with baking soda.

    Children's clothes
    De-odorizing clothes
    De-odorizing shoes
    Stain remover
    Oil remover
    De-odorize hand washables

6. Hygiene and beauty uses for baking soda.

    Homemade toothpaste
    Soak dentures, retainers, mouthguards
    Baking soda deodorant
    Mouthwash and bad breath killer
    De-product your hair
    Exfoliant scrub and hand soap

    Baking soda baths
    Dry shampoo
    Sore throat gargle

7. Personal care and health uses with baking soda.

    Baking soda antacid
    Eliminate diaper rash
    Bug bite relief
    Nasal irrigation
    Canker sore cure
    Burn relief
    Athlete's foot cure

8. Around the house with baking soda.

    Kitty litter freshener
    Carpet, mattress, and furniture freshener
    Stuffed animal freshener
    Dry shampoo for odorous pets
    Ashtray de-odorizer
    Clean floors and walls
    Fire extinguisher
    Homemade pet toothpaste

9. Baking soda outdoors.

    Car seat freshener
    Car air freshener
    Spackle substitute
    Anti-fungicide for plants
    Improve potting soil

    Septic tank
    De-icing paths
Conclusion

Introduction.

Congratulations for downloading this book – you are now one step closer to greatly improving your health, home, and hygiene from that little box of powder sitting in your fridge.

You might be asking yourself if there really are so many uses for baking soda, one of the cheapest things in your kitchen. The answer is a definitive *YES* and I'm so happy to help you discover them all. It's made a huge difference in the way that I run my household and it's light on my wallet. What more could you ask for?

What you'll find in this book is an enormous list of ways that you can maximize baking soda... and you've probably never heard of any of them. Some of them are creative, some are based on science, some are common sense, but **ALL are extremely useful and helpful**.

You'll learn health tips, cleaning tips, and hygiene tips – to say the least. You'll also see how you can apply baking soda in the kitchen, bathroom, bedroom, laundry room, and even outdoors. Yes, baking soda has uses literally everywhere inside and outside of your home. It's one of nature's great, untapped resources for your everyday use.

I expect that after reading this book, you will have a stash of baking soda in every room in your house. It's cheap, convenient, and you can get it anywhere. Now that's a motto that everyone can get behind.

Here's the Patty Korman approach to enjoying working with your home – the easier it is, the more you'll love and cherish it. These baking soda tips and tricks will help you accomplish that in no time flat. No more a chore.

Baking soda is the forgotten friend that people use for very few purposes – can you name some? I bet the only time you've ever thought about using baking soda before this book is to just put a box in your fridge.

That showcases only one of baking soda's many amazing traits. This book will teach you so many more ways you can use baking soda around your house starting **TOMORROW**.

How nice would it be to clean your house, take care of your health, and improve your hygiene with a one dollar box of powder? It's as great as it sounds and more frugal than you know.

Today is the beginning of a more productive and efficient lifestyle, brought to you by baking soda.

1. Baking soda basics.

Origins

Baking soda is a chemical compound that dates back to the days of the ancient **Egyptians**. That means it has been used for roughly 3,000 years and has stood the test of time. They used baking soda as a component in a cleaning agent that they called **natron** – even then, they recognized the inherent properties and benefits of baking soda.

Imagine that – 3,000 years ago, and people were just as innovative and creative as us. It just goes to show that the most effective products and cleaners most of the time are natural and gentle – a far cry from the harsh detergents and chemicals more commonly in use today.

Baking soda in its modern form was first created by Nicolas Leblanc in 1791, and the first commercial baking soda production factory was formed in 1846 by Austin Church and John Dwight – they created a brand that you might recognize in

Arm and Hammer. Arguably, it was used far more in the 1800s and 1900s because of the infancy of household chemicals and lack of viable options.

As we routinely reach for bleach, 409, or Comet for our purposes, we have forgotten about the general utility of baking soda. We simply don't know what to do with it now – we know we can scrub a couple of things with it, and we know that a box in the refrigerator can reduce some odors.

But did you know that you can actually consume it in small quantities (extremely safely) and mix it with other compounds for beneficial chemical reactions?

That's right – you can replace the majority of the commercial cleaners that you have under your sink, and thank goodness because the best part about baking soda is that it is safe.

Baking soda avoids all the potential harm and risk of most commercial cleaning products on the shelves of a grocery store **because it's natural**.

Most cleaning products that you can buy from markets today contain many harmful toxins, and can even be dangerous to inhale or use in small rooms. Try cleaning a bathroom with bleach while the door is closed and tell me you don't have a headache. In fact, a headache will be the least of your problems if you do this on a long-term basis.

They'll have at least some of the following chemicals: phthalates, perchloroethylene, 2-butoxyethanol, chlorine, and ammonia. If those sound evil and ominous, it's because they are. When used in excess, they can even cause lung damage and cancer.

Other side effects include:

1. Damaged skin from prolonged exposure (even from fumes!)
2. Damaged organs from skin exposure
3. Dizziness and headaches
4. Liver and kidney damage
5. Throat irritation
6. Swelling in the throat and mouth
7. Chemical burns in the esophagus and sinuses

And let's not forget that if you mix ammonia with bleach, you create a chlorine gas that is fatal within minutes. Any time you're exposing yourself to these harmful chemicals is a risk to your health.

It's like taking a horse tranquilizer to sleep instead of a normal over the counter sleeping pill. It's just unnecessary if you have better, safer options.

We can do better. With baking soda, we can avoid these dangerous side effects and stay natural all the way.

Just how does baking soda work?

The reason that baking soda works as well as it does is its **chemical makeup**. It has certain traits that allow it to serve many functions while being extremely healthy and non-toxic.

First of all, baking soda is physically mild, but slightly abrasive.

What does this mean? Baking soda is gentle, but effective. It doesn't react with many other compounds so it is widely usable. It's a powder that you could mistake for flour, but unlike flour, it's abrasive and can be used to gently scrub surfaces clean. It's also water soluble, so you will always be able to wash any excess away.

Second, baking soda neutralizes pH levels.

Baking soda is basic. It is alkaline. This means it neutralizes the natural acidity in many things, which lengthens their lives and allows them to last longer. For example, if you were to use baking soda in your plumbing and pipes, it would be able to neutralize the pH of the water and prevent corrosion of the pipes.

Now we're talking – hundreds of dollars in plumbers fees replaced by baking soda.

This applies to acidity in all walks of life, and anytime you want to manipulate the pH of something.

Third, baking soda is non-toxic.

It's natural and can even be ingested in small amounts. This makes it usable in cooking and anywhere there is the possibility of contact with skin. You can handle it safely and for extended periods of time. Baking soda is a much better alternative if you live in a small apartment, have children or pets, or just want to decrease your exposure to harmful substances. That should be everyone.

Take all of these elements and you get a substance that is amazingly versatile for use around the house.

2. Kitchen cleaning with baking soda.

Although baking soda can be used anywhere, it has the greatest utility in the kitchen.

Kitchens are gross. A kitchen always needs cleaning. A kitchen always has odors.

That's probably where the baking soda is stored in your house, so let's start there.

The kitchen is also another place where toxic and harmful cleaners are often used. For example, have you thought about what makes de-greasers effective? It's scary – imagine what that would do to your skin. There's a reason we wear gloves while cleaning the kitchen so often. Throw those out after you read this chapter on baking soda.

Bug repellent

Kitchens always attract bugs because there are odors and crumbs. Even if you're clean as can be, bugs will be in your kitchen at some point whether they are ants, beetles, or even cockroaches.

Sprinkling baking soda around areas that are prone to bugs will help keep them away. These will be areas such as under the sink, in corners, in shelves, and around where you have wet food and compost trash.

First, it inhibits the growth of mildew and mold because baking soda is a desiccant – it dries things out. Second, baking soda will absorb any leftover odors. Finally, baking soda will flat out kill bugs when they ingest it because it will create carbon dioxide in the insect and expanding their stomachs, causing them to burst.

And of course, the best part is that you can openly leave baking soda in those areas where people will be because it is safe.

Odor-killer

Odors are everywhere in your house, not just the kitchen. But the worst ones are often here because of (1) leftover food, (2) the presence of water in sinks, and (3) the garbage can overflowing with soggy matter. This can lead to bugs, and even worse – mice. If you have a small kitchen with little to not ventilation, it's going to be tough to want to step in there every day while odors are compounding.

While you can't de-odorize leftover food very well, you can definitely take care of the odors in your sinks and garbage can. In fact, you should do this quickly so layers of bacteria don't build up.

All you need to do is sprinkle baking soda over smelly areas, let it absorb the odor overnight, and wipe it away with a wet paper towel. This means you can sprinkle baking soda into the garbage can (inside the trash bag) directly, and pour it down the sink drain directly (wash down with hot water in the sink). Use liberally.

You can squeeze a lemon over the clean surfaces for an extra touch of pleasantness.

If the garbage can itself is developing an odor, you don't have to take it outside and wash it with a hose. You can also just sprinkle baking soda into the garbage can itself and it will suck up the leftover moisture and odor under the trash bag. Again, use liberally.

Fridge freshener

This is perhaps the best-known use for baking soda, and unfortunately one of the only ones that people use it for.

If you pop open a box of baking soda in your fridge, it will keep your fridge odorless. This makes it a pleasant experience for you, and it prevents strong food odors from seeping into other foods and ruining their taste.

For example, if you have something with a strong onion or garlic odor, you can prevent your entire fridge from smelling that way, and other foods from having an onion or garlic residue or taste.

Shiny surfaces

Even if you clean well, sometimes you can't avoid fingerprints on your shiny surfaces like chrome, steel, countertops, and even marble. It feels like they are unavoidable – if you clean one fingerprint, you'll leave another elsewhere.

Baking soda is a great polishing agent -- and much milder and gentler than commercial polishing agents. Recall that baking soda is a mild abrasive. This means it has the power you need.

If you polish all of these surfaces with a baking soda and water solution (1 tablespoon with 8 ounces), it will wipe away all of your fingerprints and make them shine like you never thought possible. You can also just lightly sprinkle baking soda on top of the surfaces you want to polish and wipe them down with warm paper towels.

De-odorizing bottles and flasks

I bought my husband a flask that he's used all of once because he said it just didn't feel clean after he used it once. And he's right – there's no good way to clean flasks and bottles that you can't fit a sponge or brush into.

Baking soda presents a simple solution to this.

To clean your bottles, flasks, and other utensils or containers that hold strong odors, soak them in a baking soda solution (1 tablespoon with 8 ounces of water) for an hour at a time. Rinse and repeat if necessary. Now my husband uses his flask all the time – often when it's embarrassing!

De-odorizing hands

If you have ever cooked with garlic or onions before, you know that it is difficult to get rid of odors on your hands. It doesn't matter how many times you've washed them – sometimes the odors are still there the next day.

If you cook any ethnic food at all, you'll know that this problem extends far beyond garlic and onions. How do you deal with smelly hands after you're done cooking?

You can make a simple hand scrub solution with water and baking soda (1 tablespoon with 8 ounces of water, or just sprinkle baking soda on your hands and scrub together under warm water).

An added benefit to this baking soda solution is you can quickly eliminate the odors on your hands without drying your hands out from washing them ten times.

De-odorizing sponges

We all wash our dishes with sponges, but we don't replace the sponges every day because that would be highly impractical and expensive.

However, when we keep a sponge for over a week, they start to develop an odor. And when you wash dishes, often the odor of the sponge stays on your hand instead of the soap smell.

So to eliminate this odor on the sponge, just drop your sponge into a solution of 2 tablespoons of baking soda and 16 ounces of water and let it soak for about 30 minutes. After this, you won't have to worry about a stinky sponge – for a few days anyway.

You might want to take care to sanitize your sponges daily and not just treat the odor that they cause, however.

Cleaning the microwave and oven

There are specific cleaners for both of these appliances, and they happen to be extremely harsh because of the gunk that builds up in them. This is something we want to avoid, because our food is potentially touching them. We are potentially ingesting all of those harsh chemicals I mentioned earlier when you use commercial cleaners. What if you missed a spot and some of it drips into your food directly?

Cleaning gunk in a microwave or oven is difficult because the gunk often builds up so heavily that you need to scrub vigorously before making any progress in cleaning.

Baking soda to the rescue. Here's a scrub-free method to safely clean your microwave or oven buildup.

Spread a baking soda paste of ½ cup of baking soda with ¼ cup of water, and leave it on the gunk overnight. Then in the morning, spray the baking soda with vinegar, let it bubble a bit, and wipe it all off with a damp paper towel. You can rinse and repeat if necessary with particularly tough buildups.

A side note on baking soda's reactivity with vinegar: when you combine these two substances, you create a chemical reaction because baking soda is basic and vinegar and acidic.

You might think this causes the substances to neutralize each other – this is true, but in the first few minutes following combining the two, the chemical reaction creates carbonic acid. Carbonic acid is a great cleaning agent, but is unfortunately very unstable and quickly degrades into carbon dioxide (among other things), which explains the bubbles that you'll always see. This means to effectively use baking soda and vinegar in cleaning, you cannot combine them in advance.

Mop cleaner

We use mops to clean our kitchen floors and eliminate all the splashes and drops of food waste that have fallen over weeks and months. But have you ever thought about washing the mop to make sure that you're not just spreading the filth all over the floor again?

Baking soda can help you wash your mop. Just pour ½ cup of baking soda into a bucket and soak the mop for at least 1 hour. This will be gentle on the mop, yet clean and de-odorize it.

Notably, baking soda isn't strong enough to kill the worst germs and bacteria out there, but it will eliminate the vast majority of them. To make your mop 100% clean, put a few drops of bleach into the bucket along with the baking soda.

But you must never mix bleach and vinegar, because that creates chlorine gas, which can be fatal.

Better dish soap

Sometimes our dish soap just isn't enough to cut through the grease and oil that we've used in cooking.

Health aside, we can increase the effectiveness of our dish soap if we simply sprinkle baking soda onto our sponge while we are washing dishes. It is great for cutting through grease, and makes your dish soap a bit more abrasive for better scrubbing.

3. Cooking with baking soda.

Reduce acidity in food

Baking soda is basic and a neutralizer.

This means it reduces the acidity levels of whatever it is added to. Some foods we eat are extremely acidic in terms of pH levels, which can be hard on your stomach and ultimately contribute to ulcers or acid reflux (heartburn).

Adding baking soda to the food we eat can (1) reduce tastes that are too tart, sharp, or acidic, and (2) make it easier on our stomach. That's great.

For example, you can sprinkle baking soda to tomato-based, citrus-based or vinegar-based recipes to reduce the sharp taste. Sprinkle to taste – add a little at a time until you like what you taste.

If you have actual heartburn or acid reflux problems, you can add 1 teaspoon of baking soda to 1 cup of soda and drink it slowly. This will eliminate the burning sensation and can also calm upset stomachs. Just beware if you have kidney or heart conditions, or are on certain types of medication that alter your blood pH.

De-odorizing meat

Sometimes, the meat we cook and put into our bodies has a strong, strong smell. Sometimes this is good and savory, yet other times it can still make us gag before we properly season it.

Fish and hunted game come to mind, especially.

To remove such strong odors (not spoilage, just aggressive gamey odors and flavors) from fish and hunted game, you can just let the fillets or pieces of meat soak in a tablespoon of baking soda and 16 ounces of water solution for up to an hour. Rinse the meat, and the strong odor will be gone.

Your meat will now taste much better once the edge has been removed from it. Not all of us enjoy eating meat or fish that tastes like it was just picked out from the salty ocean.

Fluffy omelets

Who's a fan of breakfast? There is no better meal in the universe. Breakfast should be had at lunch and dinner frequently.

Even if you're not a fan of breakfast in general, there is no way you won't be a fan of the fluffy, delicious omelets that baking soda can help you create. If you add ½ tablespoon of baking soda to 3 eggs and whisk it all together, your omelets will be nice and fluffy.

This creates picture-perfect omelets and also feels great in the mouth.

Easier hardboiled eggs

Hardboiled eggs can be very difficult for some people to peel. They might not have very good finger dexterity, or they are just plain bad at it.

Whatever the case, you can simplify this process by adding 2 tablespoons of baking soda to the water that you boil your eggs in. This will make the shell separate from the egg easier, and make hardboiled eggs a more accessible treat for you.

De-feathering game

If you're a hunter, you will love this tip.

Sometimes you can't be bothered to de-feather a bird by hand, and the easiest way to do it otherwise is to boil it.

Add a tablespoon of baking soda to the pot of water that you are boiling for the bird – that will help the feathers slide off easier, and keep the skin cleaner and easier to cook later. Of course, this also decreases the sometimes foul odor that comes with freshly killed meat.

Homemade Gatorade

If you have a sporting event coming up soon, you can save money by making your own Gatorade! This is easier than you think, and if you are a soccer mom and have to provide beverages for an entire team, look no further.

All you have to do is mix:

- ½ tablespoon of baking soda

- ½ tablespoon of salt
- 1 quart of water
- 1 pack of sports drink powder

After all, all sports drinks do is put sodium and salts back into athletes so they don't get dehydrated. It is a relatively simple recipe with relatively simple goals.

This can serve many kids (and adults!) for just the price of a packet of sports powder ($2.00).

Substitute for baking powder

If there are any bakers in the house, you might know what I'm talking about. Baking soda is sometimes confused with baking powder at the grocery store, and it's a completely understandable mistake.

Luckily, you can use baking soda instead of baking powder for your baking recipes, if you just mix it with cream of tartar. Two parts cream of tartar to one part baking soda.
Voila, great cake on the way. You probably won't even be able to tell that anything is different.

Tenderize meat

You can actually tenderize meat with baking soda if you have an hour to kill!
All you need to do is rub both sides of your piece of meat with baking soda, and then put it back into the fridge to wait. Make sure you coat the meat liberally with baking soda.

After about 45 minutes, simply rinse the baking soda off, and enjoy your automatically tenderized piece of meat. This works because baking soda slowly denatures the proteins in the meat that it comes in contact with.

Clean burned pans

Baking soda is really a wondrous cleaning agent – it is effective and strong, but so gentle that you can use it on almost any surface, including a non-stick Teflon frying pan.

Sometimes we're not paying attention and burn things on the stove in our pan – it's no one's fault. But how do you clean that annoying burnt matter on your pan? It might take an extreme amount of scrubbing, but that might also damage your non-stick Teflon pan.

As usual, baking soda comes to the rescue.

Boil water in the pan, and turn the stove off. Then, add about ½ cup of baking soda, depending on the size of the pan. Let this solution sit overnight. Tomorrow morning, you will be able to instantly clean the burnt matter from your pan without damaging it. Voila.

4. Bathroom upkeep with baking soda.

The next obvious place where baking soda is incredibly helpful is the bathroom. Like the kitchen, the bathroom is home to many situations where there is dirt, odor, and the need for cleaning.

Remember, baking soda will eliminate the need for harsh cleaners that can potentially be harmful to your health.

Shower curtains

You probably need to replace your shower curtains right now. Shower curtains build up bacteria and a gross residue relatively quickly, but we rarely clean them because they are just a pain in the butt. Even if you remove them from their hangers, they aren't easy to scrub because they are so flimsy.

It's often easier to just replace them.

There is an easy solution to this.

Just unhook the shower curtain from the shower curtain rod, and let it fall into the bathtub. Then fill the bathtub up with warm water and mix in 2 cups of baking soda. Stir a bit, and soak for a few hours. Rinse it off with the showerhead and your shower curtain will be shiny and good as new. No awkward scrubbing needed.

Unclogging drains

You can get around the need for harsh chemicals like Drano with baking soda.

Have you ever looked at the ingredients on a container of Drano? They are very toxic and harmful, and Drano works by literally burning away the contents of a drain clog. This is why Drano is also bad for the drains themselves.

So when you want to get rid of a blog in your drain from shaving gel or hair, all you need to do is the following.

First, pour boiling water down the drain, followed immediately by ½ cup of baking soda.

Second, combine 1 cup of vinegar with 1 cup of hot water, and pour that drain the drain. Make sure that you put the plug/stopper in to keep the chemical reaction at the clog.

Third, after letting it sit for 10 minutes, pour another pot of boiling water down the drain.

The reaction between the vinegar and baking soda is what clears the clog in your drain.

Stained toilet

If you have neglected to clean your toilet and find it stained and unpleasant to look at, baking soda can help with that. This is especially effective on hard water stains.

First, pour about 1 cup of vinegar into the toilet. Make sure it touches all the surfaces that you want to clean, above and below the water line.

Second, sprinkle about 1 cup of baking soda into the toilet. Again, make sure it touches all areas that the vinegar touched.

Watch the bubbles, then scrub lightly to achieve a clean toilet bowl.

Glass cleaner

Many of the uses I have taught you for baking soda have involved using it to scrub and get rid of buildup. It is mildly abrasive, but gentle enough so it won't harm surfaces or your skin.

This makes it ideal for glass and mirrors because baking soda isn't abrasive enough to scratch those surfaces.

To use baking soda as a cleaner for glass, mirrors, and other smooth surfaces, sprinkle a tiny bit onto a wet paper towel and just wipe the mirror with it.

Take note, you may need to wipe the glass one more time with a dry paper towel to get rid of excess baking soda, but baking soda will eliminate all oils and marks gently and effectively.

Bathroom de-odorizing

Bathrooms are notorious for unpleasant smells that are associated with bodily functions. You know what I'm talking about.

But beyond the smells that come from us, there are smells that exist because a bathroom is a damp environment. This makes it very easy for mildew, mold, fungi, and general uncleanliness to occur.

Use a box of baking soda in the bathroom as you would use it in the refrigerator. Pop it on top of the toilet, under the toilet, behind the sink, or next to the shower.

Just make sure to cover it during a shower and for about 30 minutes after so the baking soda doesn't just suck up the shower moisture.

Each box will last somewhere from 1-3 months, and will serve you well in destroying moisture and odors in your bathroom.

Floor, bathtub cleaner

This can easily go under kitchen usage of baking soda as well, but it's more common for there to be tile in the bathroom floor. And of course, porcelain tubs will benefit from this as well.

Here is all you have to do: sprinkle baking soda onto the surface that you want to clean, and then spray vinegar onto it. Let it foam and bubble for a bit, and then wipe the surface clean without having to scrub at all.

The best part is that since baking soda is so low-impact and non-toxic, your feet can touch it for hours and you will be absolutely fine. You can't say the same about any of the other cleaners that you would buy at the store! You wouldn't want to be touching those.

Toothbrush and comb freshener

Toothbrushes are actually not that clean, usually. This is half because they are used for months on end, and half because human mouths are notoriously dirty and bacteria-filled.

So if you soak your toothbrush in a solution of 4 ounces of water and ½ tablespoon of baking soda, it will de-odorize it and kill any of the remaining bacteria from your mouth. Soak it for ½ hour and enjoy the fresh feeling of a new toothbrush without having to buy one.

Of course, you can also soak your combs and brushes in baking soda without damaging them to remove excess residue and leftover product effortlessly.

Unclog showerhead

Showerheads often clog up because of a buildup of calcium in the showerhead itself. This means that half of your showerhead won't be spraying water, and it might mean that the pipes leading to the showerhead are clogged.

You may not be able to do much with the pipes unless you hire a professional, but you can fix calcium buildups in the showerhead.

All you need to do is take it off the wall and let it soak in a solution of 1 cup of vinegar and 1/3 cup of baking soda for a few hours. Add the showerhead to the vinegar first, then add the baking soda after. Make sure you cover the container as this will cause a foaming chemical reaction.

You will see the calcium slide off and rest at the bottom of the bucket, and the next time you shower you should have a full spray again.

Natural grout cleaner

As in the prior use, combining baking soda with vinegar is a great cleaner that eliminates calcium buildups. Such buildups are also extremely common in grout.
So create a paste with ½ cup of baking soda and 3-4 tablespoons of water and apply it to the grout between the tile in the shower. Then spray vinegar on top of the paste.

Let it sit for at least 30 minutes. Then scrub it lightly, and rinse off with water. The calcium should have been eliminated and your grout will be sparkly clean and white.

5. Laundry with baking soda.

We've all seen commercials where that cute bear claims that his detergent will make your clothes amazingly soft and snuggly.

He's cute, but his detergent is harsh and full of toxic chemicals. And to boot, laundry detergent is one of the more expensive cleaning agents that you can buy for your home.

So using baking soda instead of, or with your current detergent is great on many levels. Baking soda is also great for getting out stains and keeping your colors bright.

Children's clothes

Children have very delicate skin, babies especially. This leads to them getting rashes and irritated skin relatively easy.

Part of this can be traced back to the laundry detergent they use. If you are using a laundry detergent with harsh chemicals and then putting those clothes onto a baby, that's going to be difficult on their skin.

All you need to do is add ½ a cup of baking soda to the wash cycle along WITH the detergent. This will balance out the harsh chemicals of the detergent, and make them more mild but still effective as a cleaner.

De-odorizing clothes

Aside from neutralizing many of the harsh chemicals in detergent, if you sprinkle in ½ a cup of baking soda into your wash cycle with a particularly smelly load of clothes, baking soda is a great de-odorizer and your load will be fresh smelling.

You can get the hop on this by even just sprinkling some baking soda into your laundry basket to make sure that your room, or the laundry room, isn't being overtaken by the smell of some sweaty, crusty clothing.

De-odorizing shoes

Shoes stink. Feet sweat, and they stink. The sweat seeps into the shoes, and makes them stink.

Everything below your ankles is just a stink factory, but that's something that baking soda can help with.

After you take off your shoes for the day, just sprinkle a couple of tablespoons of baking soda into the shoes and shake it around a little bit to make sure it coats everything on the inside of the shoe.

Let this sit overnight. Then, just dump the baking soda out before you want to wear it next and your shoe will be much cleaner feeling and smelling. You can also do this when you want to wear your sneakers barefoot. Sprinkle 1 tablespoon into each shoe to cut down on the moisture and odor.

Stain remover

Baking soda can also be used prior to the laundry wash cycle as a stain remover. If you eat pasta and get some red sauce on your white shirt, take the shirt off immediately and apply a baking soda and water solution (2 tablespoons of baking soda and 1 tablespoon of water), let it sit for 5 minutes, then spray the stain with a mixture of equal parts water and vinegar.

Let it soak, then throw it into the wash cycle and the stain should be gone.

Oil remover

Baking soda is good at removing substances like oil and grease from objects or yourself. It soaks oil and grease up and makes it easy to deal with. This means that you can use it specifically to remove things like chapstick, lipstick, and other kinds of products from your clothes.

Just use a baking soda and water solution of equal parts of each to scrub lightly and oil-based products should come out of your clothes easily.

De-odorize hand washables

We all have delicates that we do, or should, wash by hand. Sometimes they are even so delicate that we shouldn't be using soap on them, only warm water.

The problem is that most delicates are against our skin, which means that they pick up a good amount of grease, sweat, and body odor. But if you can't use detergent… then you can use baking soda to remove all of those.

Simply add 2 tablespoons of baking soda to the sink while you are hand-washing delicates, and the odors will vanish and colors will remain bright.

6. Hygiene and beauty uses for baking soda.

Since most of health and beauty take place in the kitchen and the bathroom, this covers both of those as well!

Baking soda is an amazing agent for cleaning and de-odorizing things and objects, but it can also be amazing for cleaning yourself. The specific properties of baking soda also mean that it can help your hygiene and beauty products too.

Homemade toothpaste

You can easily use baking soda alone as a toothpaste and teeth whitener. It's cheaper than any commercial tube of toothpaste and just as safe if not safer.

You can simply sprinkle some baking soda onto your toothbrush, run it under the faucet to get it wet, and then start using it normally. Or, you can put a pinch of baking soda into a small bowl of water and combine before putting the toothbrush in your mouth.

You don't have to worry about bad breath because baking soda is great with neutralizing odors.

Many people have made a fuss about baking soda being too abrasive by itself for regular usage on teeth – but studies have shown that baking soda alone, used properly, is actually less abrasive than all commercial toothpastes. However, it's worth being careful if you have weak enamel or sensitive teeth and gums.

Soak dentures, retainers, mouthguards

Denture, retainers, and mouthguards all develop distinct odors as a result of the bacteria in your mouth over time. This is extremely unpleasant, and even a hard brushing can't always get rid of them.

No one wants to wear a stinky mouthguard, so soaking all of the above in a baking soda solution will get rid of the odor and loosen any buildup of plaque or gunk on them.

Just start with a bowl of 8 ounces of warm water, and put 1-2 tablespoons of baking soda into it and mix it. Drop your mouthguard in, and let it soak for an hour or so. When you take it out, your mouthguard will be shiny and smell like new.

Baking soda deodorant

If you're searching for a cheap, odorless way of preventing perspiration and odors from your armpits, look no further than baking soda.

All you need to do is just dust your armpits with baking soda and you will be dry and odorless all day long. Just make sure to get rid of any leftover baking soda so it doesn't look like residue from a commercial deodorant.

Mouthwash and bad breath killer

Sometimes you run out of mouthwash, or just want something odorless to freshen up your breath with. All you need to do is rinse and gargle with a cup of warm water and 1 tablespoon of baking soda.

Make sure you gargle in your throat and this solution will successfully kill the vast majority of the bacteria in your mouth.

De-product your hair

If you use hair products at all, you know that they are often hard to clean and fully get out of your hair, even when you use shampoo. And overshampooing and washing just leads to your hair and scalp drying out, which leads to dandruff… which leads to more product. It's a negative cycle.

After you squeeze your shampoo onto your palm, sprinkle a bit of baking soda into it and wash and rinse your hair as usual. The baking soda will work to bind to and remove any leftover residue of the product you have used, and clean your hair and scalp without drying it out.

Baking soda is great at removing residue and grease.

Exfoliant scrub and hand soap

Instead of buying expensive scrubs that are filled with chemicals and microbeads that are harmful to the environment and will clog your drains eventually, you can use baking soda as a scrub. Remember that baking soda is a slight abrasive.

Just make a baking soda paste from ½ cup of baking soda and ¼ cup of water, and make sure to err on the side of more baking soda so it is more solid. Scrub your face and body with it and will shed skin and become radiant after.

Baking soda baths

Instead of a bubble bath, which is prone to dry you out if you stay in it for an extended period of time, just soak in baking soda.

Run a bath and fill the tub to the level you would like, and then add 2 cups of baking soda. This will wash away dirt, perspiration from your body, and is relaxing and will leave your skin feeling moisturized and clean afterwards.

Feel free to add essential oils, potpourri, or a tiny bit of bubble bath if you want an aroma and additional sense of pleasure.

This is a process that can leave your tub clean as well if you spray the tub with vinegar after draining it a bit.

Dry shampoo

By the time we hit 5:00pm some days, our head and hair are greasy and oily from the rigors of daily life.

What do you do if you don't have time to take a complete shower? Will you be stuck with a head full of grease?

Baking soda can act as a dry shampoo because it absorbs oil and dirt easily. All you need to do is sprinkle a couple of tablespoons of baking soda into your hair, massage it through your hair and scalp in particular, and then dust your head off. Give a final look in the mirror before heading out to make sure that you don't have white powder in your hair, and enjoy your shower-free cleanliness.

Sore throat gargle

Sometimes when you develop a lump in your throat, you just know that you will be sick soon. It's a huge red flag. It makes it hard to swallow, and is probably painful during your waking hours.

If you combine 1 tablespoon of baking soda and 1 tablespoon of salt (kosher, preferably) into a glass of 8 ounces of warm water, you can use this solution to gargle with. It will help disinfect your mouth and throat, which will make your sickness milder and quicker to get over.

It will also reduce the swelling and inflammation, which will make swallowing easier and less painful.

7. Personal care and health uses with baking soda.

Baking soda has many personal care and health-related uses as well. The best part about baking soda is that it is harmless to you. You can likely never use too much baking soda on yourself, but it still has amazingly cleaning, relief, and disinfecting properties for common ailments that you might encounter.

<u>Baking soda antacid</u>

If you are prone to heartburn, you should take care to have a box of baking soda in your home at all times. This can serve you just as well as TUMS, a heartburn medicine. All you need to do is add 1 tablespoon of baking soda to 1 glass of water and drink it.

Baking soda is a neutralizer, so it will act to reduce the acid reflux you have from your stomach, eliminate heartburn, and help the core problem of indigestion in your stomach.

Be careful when ingesting baking soda as it can alter the chemical composition of your stomach if you have heart, stomach, or kidney issues.

Eliminate diaper rash

Diaper rash appears on your baby's skin as a result of being in contact with a wet diaper for too long. The rash doesn't last that long, but is definitely uncomfortable and very preventable with baking soda.

All you need to do is sprinkle some baking soda into the diaper when you put it on your child. Pay attention to where moisture will build up naturally from sweat, and from when they have an accident – these are the areas that it is more important to have baking soda around.

This soaks up the moisture and prevents diaper rash from forming in the first place. Step 1 to a happier baby.

Bug bite relief

Bug bites are one of the most annoying things in the world, and the most annoying thing about them is that you shouldn't scratch them.

Baking soda can help here. All you need to do is make a baking soda paste of ½ cup of baking soda and ¼ cup of water apply it to the itchy bite. Keep the paste on the bite for at least 15 minutes, and wash it off after.

The itchiness should be greatly decreased because the baking soda has neutralized many of the acids in the bug bite.

Repeat as often as you need – this baking soda paste is harmless and can be applied as much as you want.

Nasal irrigation

Nasal irrigation is when you use a neti pot or similar type of container to pour water into one nostril, through your sinus, and out the other nostril. It is extremely effective for dealing with allergies, sickness, and congestion.

If you have a neti pot, you can't just use water by itself. It stings the nostrils too much and makes nasal irrigation a very unpleasant experience.

What you can do is combine 1 teaspoon of baking soda with 1 teaspoon of kosher salt, and mix that with 5 ounces of warm water in your neti pot.

You will get a solution that is a fraction of the cost of store-sold solutions that is harmless and cleansing.

Canker sore cure

Canker sores are so painful because they are constantly irritated and take a while to heal.

Baking soda can help cut down on the pain associated with a canker sore and speed up the healing process.

Just make that ½ cup of baking soda and ¼ cup of water solution that you've made many times before apply it to the canker sore. Let it sit for 10 minutes, then rinse it off gently. It will relieve the pain and the sore will disappear in a matter of 1-2 days.

Burn relief

Burns are extremely painful to heal from and can take many medicines and products to properly heal without scarring.

One of the best ways to alleviate the pain from a burn is to spread a baking soda paste over it of equal parts baking soda and water, and let it sit for as long as you can. The baking soda paste is very soothing and cooling, and will dull the pain after you wash it off the burn area as well.

Do this a few times a day for burn pain relief.

Athlete's foot cure

Athlete's foot is a condition where there is literally a fungus growing on your feet and toes as a result of lack of air and ventilation in your shoes.

Baking soda is well known for its anti-fungal properties, and I've already taught you a little bit about how baking soda is a neutralizer and will alter the pH of your skin.

Put those together and baking soda can greatly help cure athlete's foot. Just soak your feet in a baking soda solution – roughly 2 cups of baking soda to a bucket of cold water to soak your feet in.

Soak your feet for 20 minutes at a time and do this twice a day to get rid of your athlete's foot naturally and quickly – without any toxic anti-fungal sprays.

8. Around the house with baking soda.

Baking soda shouldn't just be contained to the kitchen and bathroom! Baking soda has so many uses in the household that it wouldn't be a bad idea to start keeping a box in every room, bedrooms included.

Below are some of the common uses for baking soda around the house, many of which I promise you haven't even thought about before.

Kitty litter freshener

Kitty litter is notorious for stinking. After all, it's where your feline buddy relieves himself or herself, so it's to be expected. Instead of searching for a place to hide the litter box or just dealing with a stinky corner, baking soda can help de-odorize the box and freshen it up.

Just sprinkle a healthy amount of baking soda into the litter box, and even around the box on the floor to absorb the odor of the kitty litter. It's simple, easy, cheap, and makes life with your cat much more pleasurable.

Your feline friend might be confused at first, but they will adapt quickly.

Carpet, mattress, and furniture freshener

Baking soda has wonderful de-odorizing properties.

If you just leave baking soda in the presence of something stinky, then it will absorb the odor in no time at all.
Carpets, mattresses, and furniture are all things that develop odor over time. It can be a huge process to thoroughly clean those, and you might have to even rent machines to do it. Not cheap or easy.

Here's a tip – sprinkle baking soda over your carpets, mattresses, and furniture to freshen up their scent and remove any odors. Rub and massage the baking soda in.

Leave the baking soda in overnight (at least), then vacuum up the remainder. What's left is a fresh and clean smelling couch or carpet.

Just make sure that you vacuum up all the baking soda.

P.S. You can also sprinkle baking soda into purses that haven't been used in a while to get rid of their musty odors.

Stuffed animal freshener

Let's face it, you love 'em, but your kids can be stinkmonsters.

But using the same process as above – sprinkling and vacuuming – you can freshen up your child's stuffed animals and plush toys overnight. No more smell of spit, saliva, or regurgitated pasta.

You can do this more easily by putting stuffed animals or other objects into a plastic bag, putting baking soda into the bag, and sealing the bag overnight and shaking it a bit.

Dry shampoo for odorous pets

It can be a struggle to get your pet into a shower or bath. Baking soda makes freshening up your pet's scent incredibly easy.

Just treat the baking soda as dry shampoo. Sprinkle it all over your pet, and massage it through his fur and make sure you work it into his skin, which is where the oil comes from.

Leave it on your pet for as long as he can stand it, or 1 hour, and then brush your pet vigorously to get rid of the excess white baking soda powder.

Say goodbye to perpetual wet dog smell.

Ashtray de-odorizer

If you smoke indoors, you probably use an ashtray. Ashtrays can build up incredibly strong smells after time, and this isn't always pleasant to be near even if you are an avid smoker.

We know that baking soda is a wonderful de-odorizer, so to neutralize some of the smell of that ashtray, just sprinkle some baking soda into it before, during, and after you use it. It will suck up the smell of smoke in no time at all and control the odors in your home.

Clean floors and walls

To clean your floors and walls, simply make a baking soda paste, with equal parts baking soda and warm water. Use that to scrub your hardwood floors and walls without any fear of any toxic chemicals eroding them.

This is especially important when cleaning painted walls, because some cleaners may strip the paint from your walls! Baking soda is 100% harmless yet effective, so you don't have to worry about the safety of any paint.

Fire extinguisher

Obviously, this use must come with a disclaimer. If you're worried about fires, you really should obtain a fire extinguisher for your kitchen or garage. In fact, it is a good rule of thumb to have 1 per household, and check regularly to make sure that they haven't expired.

That said, baking soda can work in a pinch to put out small fires, especially those in the kitchen! If you've got a fire, simply dump baking soda over it, covering the whole fire. This will NOT increase the fire, as sugar or other powders will.

The reason this works is that baking soda produces carbon dioxide when exposed to heat, and carbon dioxide displaces the oxygen that the fire requires to burn.
But again, you should have a fire extinguisher on hand.

You should be aware that putting water on many types of fires (like oil fires) can actually make them worse, so baking soda can be used instead of water sometimes.

Homemade pet toothpaste

If you have a pet, you'll know that they get some serious kibble breath sometimes. This just gets worse when you don't brush their teeth on a regular basis – but some pets absolutely hate it, so it's difficult to police.

A big part of that is the odor and flavor of many pet toothpastes. Baking soda can substitute in a pinch for a great toothpaste as it is abrasive yet gentle – and it is odorless! Your pet will barely know what's going on because it is so gentle and it's harmless – they can even swallow it if they want, without having to rinse! Just dip your pet's toothbrush into some baking soda, wet it, and go to town.

You just have to get them to sit still for their brushing session, and that's no small feat.

9. Baking soda outdoors.

Baking soda is versatile and rough enough to be effective for outdoor uses as well. Don't think that just because baking soda is gentle that it won't be strong enough for the big, bad outdoors.

Here are some really useful and helpful uses for baking soda outside of the house.

Car seat freshener

Just like with before, it is fully possible to use baking soda to completely de-odorize your car. All you need to do is sprinkle baking soda onto the seats and floor of your car generously.

Leave it overnight, then vacuum up the excess baking soda the next day. Your car will be fresh as the day you bought it, minus the leather smell.

This works great to absorb and clean up any oil or grease spills inside the car as well.

Car air freshener

Most air fresheners that hang in our cars smell incredibly artificial. They don't even eliminate any odors that are in the car, and just mask them with a strong pine scent.

Instead of hanging a little green tree from your rearview window, try pouring some baking soda out into a deep cup, and leaving that in your drink holder. This will de-odorize your car, and should be good for about a month before changing it. You can even tape a piece of paper over the top of the cup and just poke some holes in it to make sure that the baking powder doesn't spill.

It's the car equivalent of what you do with the box of baking soda in your refrigerator.

Spackle substitute

Spackle is a substance used to fill in holes and small dents in white colored walls. Its purpose is just to make it appear aesthetically as if nothing had happened.

Unfortunately, we don't always have spackle on hand, even though it might just take a tiny bit to make something look much better.

Just make a thick baking soda paste – much thicker than any you've used before from this book, 1 cup of baking soda to ¼ cup of water. Use a broad surface like a flat metal spatula to fill in the holes and the dents, and just let it dry!

If you're feeling creative and brave, you can mix food coloring into this to attempt to fill in holes and dents in differently colored walls.

Anti-fungicide for plants

If you make a ½ cup of baking soda and 1 cup of water solution and spray it over your plants, it will make them more resistant to fungus. This combines the gentle nature of baking soda with its anti-fungal properties.

This has the added benefit of protecting your plants from insects, because as covered before, insects will die when they ingest baking soda.

Improve potting soil

Baking soda is naturally neutral and an alkaline. This means that it can lower the acidity level of soil, and this is great for plants because high levels of acid are bad for them.

This means that you can pour a 1 tablespoon baking soda and 8 ounces of water solution directly into the soil of plants to balance the pH level of the soil and it will improve the health of your houseplants. You have to make sure to do this very sparingly though, because soil that is too basic is also not healthy.

You can determine the pH of your soil easily with kits from garden stores.

De-greaser

Baking soda is an excellent de-greaser, as you already know from how baking soda can be useful in the kitchen.

But there is grease outside of the kitchen too. For example, if you have a car or motorcycle. These things leak grease and oil constantly, and sometimes you have to clean it up or prevent a buildup elsewhere.

You can simply make a ½ cup of baking soda and ½ cup of water paste and spread that onto the pile of grease or oil. It will help absorb it some, and make it much easier to grab and clean up from the car or garage floor.

Septic tank

If you add 1 cup of baking soda to your septic tank a week, it will help maintain a balanced pH level, which helps it flow better and prevents corrosion of the tank and associated pipes.

De-icing paths

When winter rolls around, often the outdoor paths we use around our homes are slippery and dangerous because of ice.

Baking soda can serve the same purpose as rock salt or kitty litter – it will provide traction over dangerous icy spots and actually melt the ice. Sprinkle it liberally over the icy parts, ideally before you have to use them.

It doesn't melt ice quite as well as rock salt, but it can work in a pinch to make your days safer.

Conclusion

I hope I've shown you many wonderful ways that baking soda can help you run your home cheaply and naturally.

I have no doubt that you will save lots of money on toxic substances like cleaners that you'll never need again. Humans didn't need Windex until about 50 years ago – we can function amazingly with natural cures and homemade remedies that involve baking soda.

I hope that you have found some value in this book, and see reason to stash a few boxes of baking soda in your home from now on.

I wish you the best,
Patty ☺

Printed in France by Amazon
Brétigny-sur-Orge, FR